Raising Your Baby Green:

How to Start A Earth-Friendly Family

I0411730

Teagan Smith

Table of Contents

Chapter 1:

Why be Earth-friendly

The inhabitants of this planet are among the luckiest of all creatures, as they have one of the best places to live. Making this comparison may seem illogical to many, yet scientists believe that this universe is so diverse that it surely has unlimited plants and living spaces. Earth is a unique situation as it possesses everything which is needed to keep human life living.

We always talk about transitions and changes which have taken place from the beginning of time until now. One thing which has remained the same is where we as humans have lived, Earth. No matter how advanced human civilisation has become, mankind cannot change where it lives. Earth is an irreplaceable resource for the wellbeing of humankind. Unfortunately, mankind has not always been kind to the world it lives in. We need to start being aware of what our responsibilities are as a world village are in order to save this Planet for future generations!

What does it mean to be Earth-friendly?

Being Earth-friendly refers to an attitude of being friendly and responsible to nature and its wellbeing. Earth is the only planet that can sustain human life. We need to be environmentally friendly in order to protect our world and all it holds. The matter is not just about protecting the Earth but also improving it as well. An environmentally friendly person makes their living habits transformed in a way that is best for the Earth and for its children.

Being Earth-friendly is now no longer an option but now is a necessity. We all need to play our part, both individually as well as collectively, to make earth an even better place to live.

> **We do not have any other options**

Being an inhabitant of this earth you need to think not just about yourself but about coming generations. Maybe your life will pass without any major changes but your grandchildren and great-grandchildren will have to pay for the decisions we are making as a group today.

> **Even technology cannot save the Earth**

Modern man is over-relying on technology. From minor tasks of everyday life to large scientific operations, everything is driven by technology. Technology has yet not given us an alternative to live in some other place. Think of the unique combination of physical properties of the earth along with its chemical combination. This makes the Earth the only place where we can enjoy a pleasurable life.

Chapter 2:

During pregnancy tips

Being earth-friendly does not necessarily mean that you need to lead a large campaign to protect the earth. Every individual can play their part by having an awareness that the prosperity of the earth lies in our awareness of the role which we can play in conserving its beauty. We have been repeatedly mentioning the need for individual contribution. You may be curious as to what one can do to start the process of changing the Earth. You're about to read about one of the first thing that anyone can do.

Green babies

There's no need for alarm – we're not talking about babies that actually the color green. "Green Baby" is a symbolic term. A "green baby" is a child whose birth, parenting, and upbringing have been carried out in a way that is not harmful to the environment and the earth. The actual concept of "green baby" means that we need to nurture the habits of being earth-friendly from the very beginning of one's life.

Raising green babies will create communities that are collectively as well as individually aware about the need of being earth-friendly. When a child is looked after in an earth-friendly way, they will have a more natural bend towards taking care of this earth.

Pregnancy tips for ensuring a green baby

If you are determined to raise a green baby then you need to start this venture from the first day that you find out that a new little one is coming into your life.

Here are some guidelines for those who want to have a green pregnancy.

The greenest place, the womb

Being pregnant, you are now in charge of two souls. Your little one is too vulnerable to face this world and its harsh realities by itself. That is the reason why nature has arranged for a better place for this little one, which is the womb. It is our responsibility to make the womb the safest and the greenest place. Take care of yourself and be careful of what you bring into your body as the smallest harmful things can make the greatest different to a green pregnancy.

Eating green – now you are not alone

Start researching now how to create a healthier diet. Junk food, pre-packaged food and processed food are no longer going to cut it. Stay away from soda, pop, and all caffeinated beverages. Eat as much organic food as you can. Drink plenty of fresh juices that are made with raw green leafy vegetables. They are packed full of the nutrients that you need.

Exercising- it's healthy

Many people quit exercise when they find out they are expecting. It is recommended to keep going with exercise, however. It can make for an easier delivery and fight fatigue during pregnancy as well. It is also a way to improve sleeping habits as well.

Make your surrounding green and clean

During pregnancy you will encounter abrupt physical and emotional changes and yes, there will be frequent mood swings. There will be times when you will be feeling depressed for no reason. One of the most crucial factors during pregnancy is to keep your surroundings positive. Get as many trees around you as you can. It will add to the positivity of your pregnancy. Additionally, keep your surroundings clean and aromatic. Take the garbage out as quickly as you can and make sure you are using materials that can be completed or recycled.

Chapter 3:
Delivery and post-delivery tips

Raising a green baby is not just about thinking about change but implementing the lifestyle that will bring about change. The basic theme of the green baby movement is to raise children who are sensitive towards the earth and its natural resources. These babies, when nurtured in an earth friendly way, will ultimately struggle for the beauty of this earth. They will eventually grow up into responsible citizens and will work for the safety of their planet. Therefore, every stage of the baby's life cycle must be focused on green and earth friendly habits and procedures.

Even the delivery and the post-delivery events are highly sensitive in raising green babies and one cannot keep themselves careless about these crucial phases of raising green babies. Some of the most helpful tips for ensuring earth friendly behaviours and attitudes are as follows:

The choice of hospital and the delivery staff

Even if you are not interested or aware of raising green babies, you need to be very selective in the choice of the hospital for the delivery procedure. Select a hospital which is producing less pollution and which is adding towards the safety of this planet. Many hospitals rely on potentially harmful medicines and use materials which are dumped directly into the environment without any concern. The doctors and staff play an important rule in your mission. If any of them are unaware of their responsibility towards the planet it can hinder your dream of raising a green baby. Select where will be the baby delivered and who will deliver the baby only after much research and deliberation.

Don't discount a mid-wife

A trend in pregnancy currently is the mid-wife and birthing center. People are starting to thoroughly enjoy this option as it gives them more control over the journey of their little one into the world. Harmful chemicals are not used and the bonding time between the parent and the baby is allowed to be as natured intended it. Highly consider looking into the mid-wife and birth center option as it could be the greenest option of all when it comes to having a green baby.

The post-delivery concerns

> You may need to stay in the hospital for a day or two after the delivery. These days are highly crucial regarding your green baby. Ask for a room from where you can easily have fresh air along with some

small trees or plants. Another benefit of having a birth-center delivery is that you are usually able to return to your home the same day.

➢ Make sure that you use all organic products during the recovery phase. All your body lotions and other personal care products must be made up of organic materials. Do not go for artificial energy drinks with dozens of chemicals and additives. If you are feeling low on energy then go for natural products such as fresh fruits and vegetables.

➢ You must also be conscious about what you are wearing when you are handling the baby. Wear clothing that contains as many natural materials as you can. A green baby must be fed in the most natural way. Do not go for artificial milk or formula unless absolutely necessary. Choose breastfeeding so that your green baby has access to the most natural food as Mother Nature intended.

➤

Bringing your infant home in a 'green' way

After spending an initial few hours or days in medical care, there will come a time when you will be bringing your baby to your home. Even minor details mean a lot and are critical when it comes to raising a green baby. Make sure that the mode of transportation used by the parents for bringing the baby home is the least hazardous for the environment. If your car is giving out highly polluted fumes, first fix this issue.

Before the baby is home, make sure you have made the perfect green arrangements for the nursery. The room where the baby must be focused on earth-friendliness. Try to keep the temperature controlled using windows that allow for fresh air to circulate. Do not use scented air fresheners as they are usually full of chemicals and artificial additives. Use safe fabric and materials for the crib, changing table, and anything else the baby will come in contact with.

Chapter 4:
Raising your baby for a green family

Raising a baby green is not just about having a baby who is earth friendly but it is about forming the foundations for a green family as well. When all of the family members have an earth-friendly approach it will eventually make up a family unit which is contributing towards the safety of this planet. A number of these green families will make up green communities which are aware of the need for the protection of this earth. Many of these communities will ultimately result in a global family which is focused on making the world a better place.

Bringing up him/her green

➢ Make your baby sensitive towards the use of green product. One of the most frequently used baby products is the diaper. Babies use many diaper on a daily basis. The question is what to use instead of these normally harmful diapers. Make sure that the material used in the diapers is earth friendly and biodegradable. Even the act of disposing normal diapers can greatly effect the future livelihood of the earth and cause our landfills to grow even larger and larger.

➢ The in-house arrangements for raising the babies are also very critical. Many of us rely heavily on the use of chemicals and disinfectants to kill germs and infections. These can be extremely harmful to a young and developing child. Look into using home remedy solutions instead for cleaning supplies. Many of these remedies are very effective, especially if they include the use of vinegar and baking soda. The use of citric fruits also makes us more protected against bacterial infections and problems.

Consider the surroundings of the baby:

➢ Keep your house arranged in the most earth-friendly way. Avoid having unnecessary materials. Make sure that you have a specific corner in your home where there are plenty of flowers and greenery. It will create a love for nature in your baby. Set aside moments of each day in which you will spend time outside with your baby in nature. Even when they are in the infant stage, try to have them in your lap and admiring the beauty of nature. Play with flowers and plants around so that the baby can see the beauty of nature even from a small age. When they become older they can be involved in planting a garden. It will create a sense of responsibility in the baby to play his part in making his surrounding clean and beautiful. Make him a responsible inhabitant of this earth from the beginning of his life. Make him admire the beauty and exclusiveness of this planet, so that he grows up to be one who wants to protect this special world.

- ➢ Make every corner of your home an earth sensitive place. Start with your kitchen as it is the place from where you feed yourself as well as your family. Make your kitchen also a place of home remedy.

- ➢ Have a small organic farm at your home. Even a small kitchen farm will be enough for a family of average size.

Use all natural soil and be cautious of using things such as fertilizer or quick grow solutions.

Chapter 5:
Raising a whole green family

In the beginning, we have discussed that earth is the most beautiful and the most secure place for the survival of mankind. Even the miracles of technology cannot bring another planet which can sustain human life. When we will start incorporating our individual contribution to make this earth green and secure it will eventually make a better earth which is free of hazardous and disastrous effects. Although we are divided in little family units, we start to belong to a global family that is focused on protecting the earth.

When you will be able to raise the green baby you will be adding a green member to your family. When all the members are sensitive to keep the earth secure and safe it will potentially benefit all other members. Green families are a true blessing for this planet, which can easily eliminate the hazardous effects of modern civilisation and a number of different pollution factors. In the larger context, these green families can unite to guide all others, so that we can fully eradicate this phenomenon of earth pollution and destruction. Eventually it will help us cherish and desire a safer planet.

➢ Recycling habit of the family

To be a sensible and green citizen, you need to avoid unnecessarily throwing things away. Try to develop a recycling habit in your family members, even including the green baby. Recycling is not only related to the disposal of materials, but it also entails that we use these materials to their full usable life. Using the materials once or twice and then disposing of them has become a common trend of modern man. It must be minimized, especially by those who are determined to raise green babies and green families. Look into making a compost pile in the backyard which can help with your unwanted materials as well. Recycling is the easiest method of making this planet safe and secure. Make recycling a daily habit of your family, so that you can truly make an earth friendly and green family.

➢ Power consumption habits of the family

From the lightning systems to the cooling and heating system, all of our power generation effect the cleanliness of this planet in one way or the other. First of all, our dependence on the artificial cooling and heating systems has made us addicted to using artificial means to survive the harsh climates, whether it is hot or cold. However, it is more conducive to use warm cloths and warm food items during the cold seasons rather than having large heating systems in our homes. Also, the construction of a home can be planned in such a way so that fresh air can come into the home and greatly reduce the need for a central air ventilation system. Minimize the use of unnecessary lights in your home as well so to conserve energy which also helps your electricity bill.

➢ Mode of transportation

One of the major reasons for the destruction of the natural environment of this planet is the over reliance and extra usage of transportation. The roads are full of vehicles and automobiles. We have increased our reliance on these vehicles so much that the physical activity has almost become invisible in the modern civilization. Even a few miles travelled through using heavy automobiles consume large amounts of fuel. It is not only a waste of natural resources like petroleum but also a cause of increased pollution on this planet. When you are nurturing a green family make sure that you incorporate a habit of physical exercise and healthy physical activity so that not only the use of an automobile can be reduced but the physical health can also be enhanced. Even when you are using an automobile for long distance travel, make it green and earth-friendly. Check the fuel consumption services of your automobile frequently so that it may not be consuming too much fuel.

All these little but important steps will eventually raise generations and communities which will be conscious towards the safety of this planet.